What I need to know about Bladder Control for Women

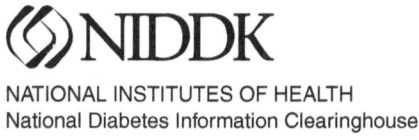

NATIONAL INSTITUTES OF HEALTH
National Diabetes Information Clearinghouse

Contents

*Inserts in back pocket

    A. What Your Doctor Needs to Know

    B. Your Daily Bladder Diary

    C. Kegel Exercise Tips

    D. Medicines for Bladder Control

Urine Leakage: A Common Health Problem for Women of All Ages

You may think bladder control problems are something that happen when you get older. The truth is that women of all ages have urine leakage. The problem is also called incontinence. Men leak urine too, but the problem is more common in women.

- Many women leak urine when they exercise, laugh hard, cough, or sneeze.

- Often women leak urine when they are pregnant or after they have given birth.

- Women who have stopped having their periods—menopause—often report bladder control problems.

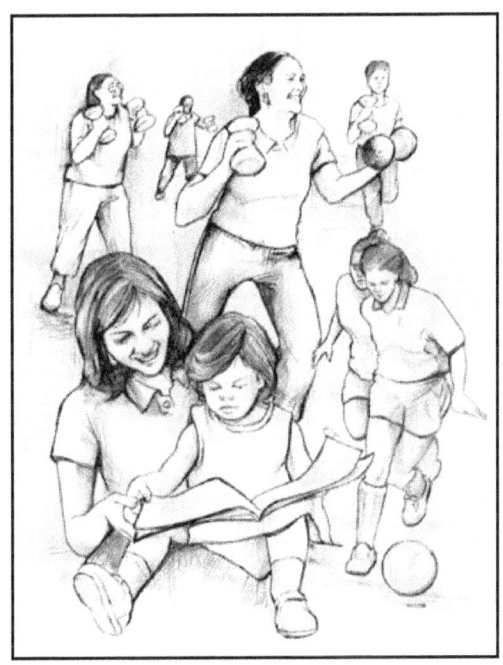

- Female athletes of all ages sometimes have urine leakage during strenuous sports activities.

Women of all ages have bladder control problems.

Urine leakage may be a small bother or a large problem. About half of adult women say they have had urine leakage at one time or another. Many women say it's a daily problem.

Urine leakage is more common in older women, but that doesn't mean it's a natural part of aging. You don't have to "just live with it." You can do something about it and regain your bladder control.

Incontinence is not a disease. But it may be a sign that something is wrong. It's a medical problem, and a doctor or nurse can help.

How does the bladder work?

The bladder is a balloon-shaped organ that stores and releases urine. It sits in the pelvis. The bladder is supported and held in place by pelvic muscles. The bladder itself is a muscle.

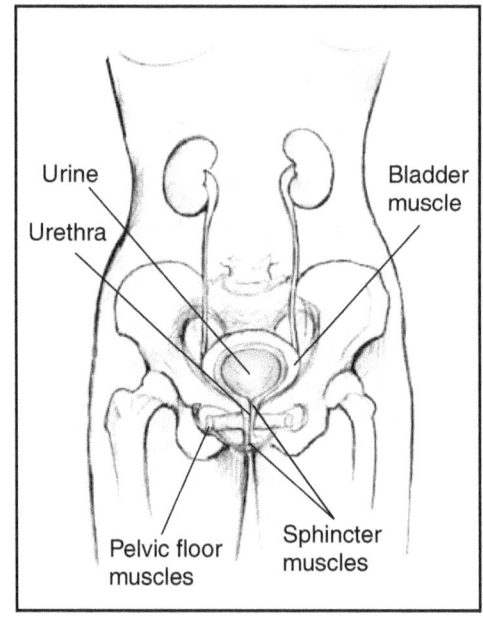

Parts of the bladder control system.

The tube that carries urine from your body is called the urethra. Ring-like muscles called sphincters help keep the urethra closed so urine doesn't leak from the bladder before you're ready to release it.

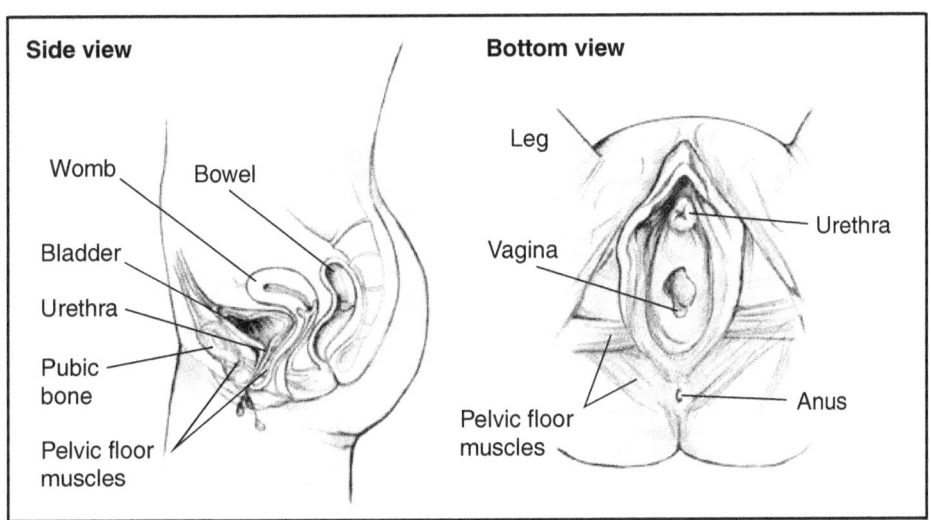

Side view	Bottom view
Womb	Leg
Bowel	
Bladder	Urethra
Urethra	Vagina
Pubic bone	Anus
Pelvic floor muscles	Pelvic floor muscles

Parts of the bladder control system.

Several body systems must work together to control the bladder.

- Pelvic floor muscles hold the bladder in place.

- Sphincter muscles keep the urethra closed.

- The bladder muscle relaxes when it fills with urine and squeezes when it's time to urinate.

- Nerves carry signals from the bladder to let the brain know when the bladder is full.

- Nerves also carry signals from the brain to tell the bladder when it's time to urinate.

- Hormones help keep the lining of the bladder and urethra healthy.

Bladder control problems can start when any one of these features is not working properly.

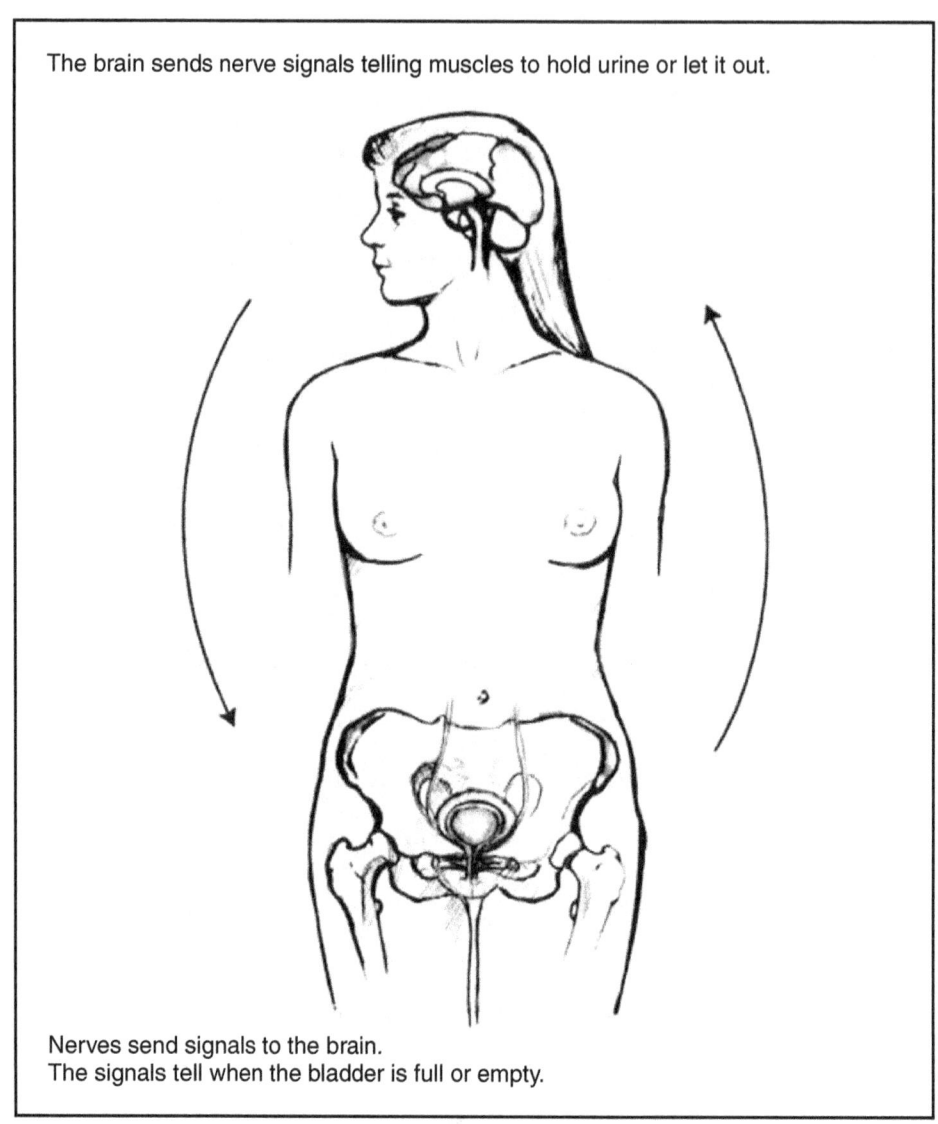

The brain sends nerve signals telling muscles to hold urine or let it out.

Nerves send signals to the brain.
The signals tell when the bladder is full or empty.

Parts of the bladder control system: nerves and brain.

4

What are the different types of bladder control problems?

Not all bladder control problems are alike. Some problems are caused by weak muscles, while others are caused by damaged nerves. Sometimes the cause may be a medicine that dulls the nerves.

To help solve your problem, your doctor or nurse will try to identify the type of incontinence you have. It may be one or more of the following six types.

- **Temporary incontinence.** As the name suggests, temporary incontinence doesn't last. You may have an illness, like a urinary tract infection, that causes frequent and sudden urination that you can't control. Or you may find that a new medicine has the unexpected side effect of increasing your urination. These problems go away as soon as the cause is found and corrected.

- **Stress incontinence.** If you leak urine when you cough, laugh, sneeze, or exercise, you have stress incontinence. Mental stress does **not** cause stress incontinence. The "stress" is pressure on the bladder. When your pelvic and sphincter muscles are strong, they can handle the extra pressure from a cough, sneeze, exercise, or laugh. But when those muscles are weak, that sudden pressure can push urine out of the bladder.

In stress incontinence, weak pelvic muscles can let urine escape when a cough or other action puts pressure on the bladder.

- **Urge incontinence.** If you leak urine after a strong, sudden urge to urinate, you have urge incontinence. This bladder control problem may be caused by nerve damage from diabetes, a stroke, an infection, or another medical condition.

- **Mixed incontinence.** Mixed incontinence is a mix of stress and urge incontinence. You may leak urine with a laugh or sneeze at one time. At another time, you may have a sudden, uncontrollable urge to urinate just before you leak.

- **Functional incontinence.** Some people have trouble getting to the bathroom. If you have urine leakage because you can't walk or have other mobility problems, you have functional incontinence.

- **Overactive bladder.** If you have to urinate eight or more times a day, you may have an overactive bladder. Getting up to urinate two or more times each night is another sign of overactive bladder. With an overactive bladder, you feel strong, sudden urges to urinate, and you also may have urge incontinence.

What causes bladder control problems?

Urine leakage has many possible causes.

- **Weak muscles.** Most bladder control problems are caused by weak pelvic muscles. These muscles may become stretched and weak during pregnancy and childbirth. Weak muscles let the bladder sag out of position, which may stretch the opening to the urethra.

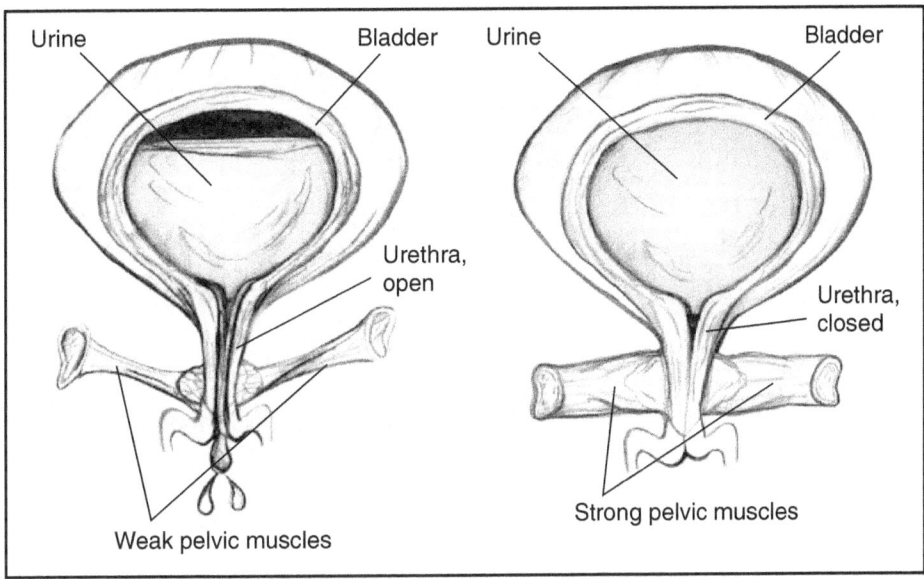

Weak pelvic muscles and strong pelvic muscles.

- **Nerve damage.** Damaged nerves may send signals to the bladder at the wrong time. As a result, a bladder spasm may push out urine without warning. Sometimes damaged nerves send no signals at all, and the brain can't tell when the bladder is full. Nerves can be damaged by diseases or trauma.

7

Diseases and conditions that can damage the nerves include

- diabetes
- Parkinson's
- multiple sclerosis
- stroke

Trauma that can damage the nerves includes

- pelvic or back surgery
- herniated disc
- radiation

- **Medicines, alcohol, and caffeine.** Leaking can happen when medicines affect any of the muscles or nerves. You may take medicine to calm your nerves so that you can sleep or relax. This medicine may dull the nerves in the bladder and keep them from signaling the brain when the bladder is full. Without the message and urge, the bladder overflows. Drinking alcohol can also cause these nerves to fail. Water pills—diuretics—take fluid from swollen areas of your body and send it to the bladder. This rapid filling may cause the bladder to leak. Caffeine drinks such as coffee and cola also cause the bladder to fill quickly. Make sure your drinks are decaf.

- **Infection.** A urinary tract infection can irritate bladder nerves and cause the bladder to squeeze without warning. This type of incontinence goes away once the infection has been cured.

- **Excess weight.** Being overweight can put pressure on the bladder and contribute to stress incontinence.

How do I tell my health care team about my urine leakage?

Talking about bladder control problems is not easy for some people. You may feel embarrassed to tell your doctor. But talking about the problem is the first step in finding an answer. Also, you can be sure your doctor has heard it all before. You will not shock or embarrass your doctor or nurse.

Medical History

You can prepare for your visit to the doctor's office by gathering the information your doctor will need to understand your problem. Make a list of the medicines you are taking. Include prescription medicines and those you buy over the counter, like aspirin or antacid. List the fluids you drink regularly, including sodas, coffee, tea, and alcohol. Tell the doctor how much of each drink you have in an average day.

Finding a Doctor

You will need to find a doctor who is skilled in helping women with urine leakage. If your primary doctor shrugs off your problem as normal aging, for example, ask for a referral to a specialist—a urogynecologist or a urologist who specializes in treating female urinary problems. You may need to be persistent, or you may need to look to organizations to help locate a doctor in your area. See pages 18 and 19 for a list of organizations.

Make a note of any recent surgeries or illnesses you have had. Let the doctor know how many children you have had. These events may or may not be related to your bladder control problem.

Finally, keep track of the times when you have urine leakage. Note what you were doing at the time. Were you coughing, laughing, sneezing, or exercising? Did you have an uncontrollable urge to urinate when you heard running water?

You can use the *What Your Doctor Needs to Know* (Insert A) and *Your Daily Bladder Diary* (Insert B) included with this booklet to prepare for your appointment.

Physical Exam

The doctor will give you a physical exam to look for any health issues that may be causing your bladder control problem. Checking your reflexes can show possible nerve damage. You will give a urine sample so the doctor can check for a urinary tract infection. For women, the exam may include a pelvic exam. Tests may also include taking an ultrasound picture of your bladder. Or the doctor may examine the inside of your bladder using a cystoscope, a long, thin tube that slides up into the bladder through the urethra.

Bladder Function Tests

Your exam may include one or more tests that involve filling the bladder with warm fluid to measure the pressure at which leakage may occur. One simple test is called a stress test. You simply relax and then cough strongly to see if urine escapes.

Any medical test can be uncomfortable. Bladder testing may sound embarrassing, but the health professionals who perform the tests will try to make you feel comfortable and give you as much privacy as possible.

How is loss of bladder control treated?

Your doctor will likely offer several treatment choices. Some treatments are as simple as changing some daily habits. Other treatments require taking medicine or using a device. If nothing else seems to work, surgery may help a woman with stress incontinence regain her bladder control.

Talk with your doctor about which treatments might work best for you.

Pelvic Muscle Strengthening

Many women prefer to try the simplest treatment choices first. Kegel exercises strengthen the pelvic muscles and don't require any equipment. Once you learn how to "Kegel," you can Kegel anywhere. The trick is finding the right muscles to squeeze. Your doctor or nurse can help make sure you are squeezing the right muscles. Your doctor may refer you to a specially trained physical therapist who will teach you to find and strengthen the sphincter muscles. Learning when to squeeze these muscles can also help stop the bladder spasms that cause urge incontinence. After about 6 to 8 weeks, you should notice that you have fewer leaks and more bladder control. Use the pelvic muscle exercise log included with the *Kegel Exercise Tips* sheet (Insert C) in this booklet to keep track of your progress.

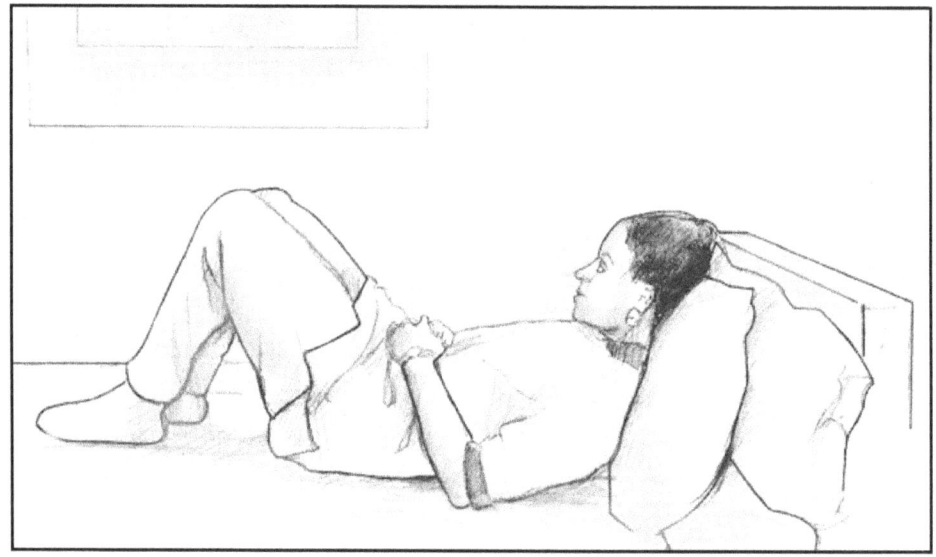

You can do Kegel exercises while lying down, sitting at a desk, or standing up.

Changing Habits

Timed voiding. By keeping track of the times you leak urine, you may notice certain times of day when you are most likely to have an accident. You can use that information to make planned trips to the bathroom ahead of time to avoid the accident. Once you have established a safe pattern, you can build your bladder control by stretching out the time between trips to the bathroom. By forcing your pelvic muscles to hold on longer, you make those muscles stronger.

Diet changes. You may notice that certain foods and drinks cause you to urinate more often. You may find that avoiding caffeinated drinks like coffee, tea, or cola helps your bladder control. You can choose the decaf version of your favorite drink. Make sure you are not drinking too much fluid because that will cause you to make a large amount of urine. If you are bothered by nighttime urination, drink most of your fluids during the day and limit your drinking after dinner. You should not, however, avoid drinking fluids for fear of having an accident. Some foods may irritate your bladder and cause urgency. Talk with your doctor about diet changes that might affect your bladder.

Weight loss. Extra body weight puts extra pressure on your bladder. By losing weight, you may be able to relieve some of that pressure and regain your bladder control.

Medicines

No medications are approved to treat stress urinary incontinence. But if you have an overactive bladder, your doctor may prescribe a medicine that can calm muscles and nerves. Medicines for overactive bladder come as pills, liquid, or a patch.

Medicines to treat overactive bladder can cause your eyes to become dry. These medicines can also cause dry mouth and constipation. If you take medicine to treat an overactive bladder, you may need to take steps to deal with the side effects.

- Use eye drops to keep your eyes moist.

- Chew gum or suck on hard candy if dry mouth bothers you. Make it sugarless gum or candy to avoid tooth decay.

- Take small sips of water throughout the day.

Medicines for other conditions also can affect the nerves and muscles of the urinary tract in different ways. Pills to treat swelling—edema—or high blood pressure may increase urine output and contribute to bladder control problems.

Talk with your doctor; you may find that taking a different medicine solves the problem without adding another prescription. The list of *Medicines for Bladder Control* (Insert D) included with this booklet will give you more information about specific medicines.

Pessaries

A pessary is a plastic ring, similar to a contraceptive diaphragm, that is worn in the vagina. It will help support the walls of the vagina, lifting the bladder and nearby urethra, leading to less stress leakage. A doctor or nurse can fit you with the best shape and size pessary for you and teach you how to care for it. Many women use a pessary only during exercise while others wear their pessary all day to reduce stress leakage. If you use a pessary, you should see your doctor regularly to check for small scrapes in the vagina that can result from using the device.

Nerve Stimulation

Electrical stimulation of the nerves that control the bladder can improve symptoms of urgency, frequency, and urge incontinence, as well as bladder emptying problems, in some people. This treatment is usually offered to patients who cannot tolerate or do not benefit from medications. At first, your doctor will use a device outside your body to deliver stimulation through a wire implanted under your skin to see if the treatment relieves your symptoms. If the temporary treatment works well for you, you may be able to have a permanent device implanted that delivers stimulation to the nerves in your back, much like a pacemaker. The electrodes in the permanent device are placed in your lower back through a minor surgical procedure.

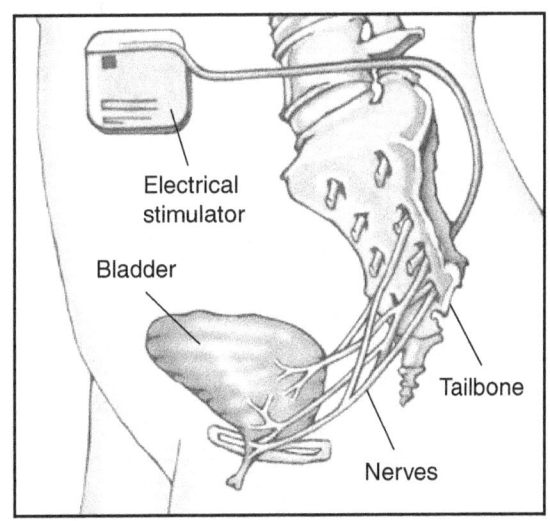

Electrical stimulator

Bladder

Tailbone

Nerves

A device can be placed under your skin to deliver mild electrical pulses to the nerves that control bladder function.

You may need to return to the doctor for adjustments to find the right setting that controls your bladder symptoms.

Surgery

Doctors may suggest surgery to improve bladder control if other treatments have failed. Surgery helps only stress incontinence. It won't work for urge incontinence. Many surgical options have high rates of success.

Most stress incontinence problems are caused by the bladder neck dropping toward the vagina. To correct this problem, the surgeon raises the bladder neck or urethra and supports it with a ribbon-like sling or web of strings attached to a muscle or bone. The sling holds up the bottom of the bladder and the top of the urethra to stop leakage.

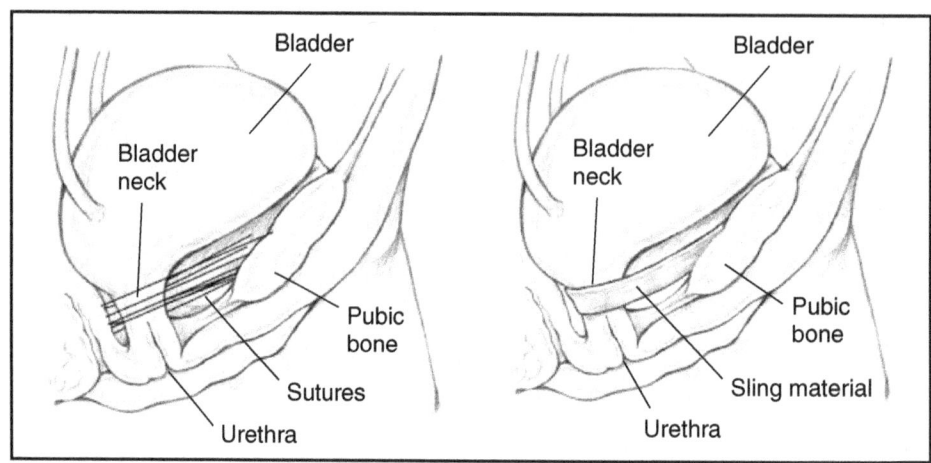

Surgery to lift the bladder may use a web of strings (left) or a ribbon-like sling (right) to support the bladder neck and urethra.

Catheterization

If your bladder does not empty well as a result of nerve damage, you might leak urine. This condition is called overflow incontinence. You might use a catheter to empty your bladder. A catheter is a thin tube you can learn to insert through the urethra into the bladder to drain urine. You may use a catheter once in a while, a few times a day, or all of the time. If you use the catheter all the time, it will drain urine from your bladder into a bag you can hang from your leg. If you use a catheter all the time, you should watch for possible infections.

Hope Through Research

The National Institute of Diabetes and Digestive and Kidney Diseases (NIDDK) supports researchers who are looking for the best ways to treat bladder control problems. The NIDDK started the Urinary Incontinence Treatment Network to gather information about the success of different treatments for bladder control problems in women. These studies will help doctors give better advice to women about the short- and long-term results and side effects of the treatments for urinary incontinence. The NIDDK has also joined a team of organizations to form the Women's Urologic Health Program. The goal of this program is to raise awareness among health care providers, patients, and the public of the advances in the treatment and prevention of women's urologic conditions to improve the quality of life for women with these conditions.

For More Information

American Urogynecologic Society
2025 M Street, NW, Suite 800
Washington, DC 20036
Phone: 202–367–1167
Email: info@augs.org
Internet: www.augs.org

American Urological Association Foundation
1000 Corporate Boulevard
Linthicum, MD 21090
Phone: 1–800–828–7866 or 410–689–3700
Fax: 410–689–3998
Email: auafoundation@auafoundation.org
Internet: www.UrologyHealth.org

National Association for Continence
P.O. Box 1019
Charleston, SC 29402–1019
Phone: 1–800–BLADDER (252–3337) or 843–377–0900
Email: memberservices@nafc.org
Internet: www.nafc.org

The Simon Foundation for Continence
P.O. Box 815
Wilmette, IL 60091
Phone: 1–800–23–SIMON (237–4666) or 847–864–3913
Email: simoninfo@simonfoundation.org
Internet: www.simonfoundation.org

Society of Urologic Nurses and Associates
P.O. Box 56
East Holly Avenue
Pitman, NJ 08071–0056
Phone: 1–888–TAP–SUNA (827–7862) or 856–256–2335
Email: suna@ajj.com
Internet: www.suna.org

Acknowledgments

The National Kidney and Urologic Diseases Information Clearinghouse (NKUDIC) would like to thank the following individuals for assisting with the scientific and editorial review of this publication.

Toby Chai, M.D.
University of Maryland

Charles Nager, M.D.
University of California, San Diego

Halina Zyczynski, M.D.
University of Pittsburgh

Thank you also to Vicki McClelland, executive director of the Free Medical Clinic of the Northern Shenandoah Valley in Winchester, VA, for facilitating field-testing of this publication.

National Kidney and Urologic Diseases Information Clearinghouse

3 Information Way
Bethesda, MD 20892–3580
Phone: 1–800–891–5390
Fax: 703–738–4929
Email: nkudic@info.niddk.nih.gov
Internet: www.kidney.niddk.nih.gov

The National Kidney and Urologic Diseases Information Clearinghouse (NKUDIC) is a service of the National Institute of Diabetes and Digestive and Kidney Diseases (NIDDK). The NIDDK is part of the National Institutes of Health of the U.S. Department of Health and Human Services. Established in 1987, the Clearinghouse provides information about diseases of the kidneys and urologic system to people with kidney and urologic disorders and to their families, health care professionals, and the public. The NKUDIC answers inquiries, develops and distributes publications, and works closely with professional and patient organizations and Government agencies to coordinate resources about kidney and urologic diseases.

Publications produced by the Clearinghouse are carefully reviewed by both NIDDK scientists and outside experts.

This publication may contain information about medications used to treat a health condition. When this publication was prepared, the NIDDK included the most current information available. Occasionally, new information about medication is released. For updates or for questions about any medications, please contact the U.S. Food and Drug Administration at 1–888–INFO–FDA (463–6332), a toll-free call, or visit their website at *www.fda.gov.* Consult your doctor for more information.

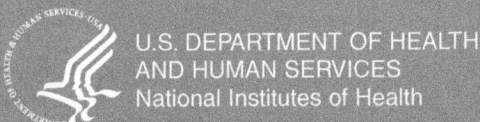

U.S. DEPARTMENT OF HEALTH
AND HUMAN SERVICES
National Institutes of Health

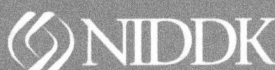

National Institute of Diabetes and
Digestive and Kidney Diseases

NIH Publication No. 07–4195
August 2007

What Your Doctor Needs to Know

To prepare for your doctor's appointment, check all the boxes below that apply to you. This information will help your doctor understand your bladder control problem.

❑ I take these prescription medicines:

medicine: _____ dose: _____

medicine: _____ dose: _____

medicine: _____ dose: _____

❑ I take these over-the-counter drugs (such as Tylenol, aspirin, or Maalox):

medicine: _____ dose: _____

medicine: _____ dose: _____

medicine: _____ dose: _____

If you take more medicines, please list them on a separate paper.

I started having bladder trouble
    ❑ within the past few months
    ❑ 1 to 2 years ago
    ❑ _____ years ago

❑ Number of babies I have had: _____
Dates: _____

❑ My periods have stopped—menopause.
Date: _____

❑ I had an operation.
Date: _____
Type of operation: _____

National Kidney and Urologic Diseases Information Clearinghouse • 1–800–891–5390
www.kidney.niddk.nih.gov

❑ I recently hurt myself or have been sick.
Date: _____
Type of injury or illness: _____

❑ I recently had a bladder—urinary tract—infection.
Date: _____

❑ I smoke cigarettes.

❑ I have pain or a burning feeling when I urinate.

❑ I often have a *really* strong urge to urinate right away.

❑ Sometimes my bladder feels full, even after I finish urinating.

❑ I go to the bathroom often, but very little urine comes out.

❑ I don't go out with friends or family because I worry about leaking urine.

❑ The first thing I do at new places is check the bathroom location.

❑ I worry about being put in a nursing home because of bladder control problems.

I have, or had, these medical problems:

❑ cancer   ❑ depression

❑ crippling arthritis   ❑ diverticulitis

❑ diabetes   ❑ multiple sclerosis

❑ interstitial cystitis   ❑ stroke

❑ spinal cord injury   ❑ other_____

❑ urinary infection

Your Daily Bladder Diary

This diary will help you and your health care team figure out the causes of your bladder control trouble. The "sample" line shows you how to use the diary.

Your name: _____

Date: _____

Time	Drinks		Trips to the Bathroom		Accidental Leaks	Did you feel a strong urge to go?	What were you doing at the time?
	What kind?	*How much?*	*How many times?*	*How much urine? (circle one)*	*How much? (circle one)*	*Circle one*	*Sneezing, exercising having sex, lifting, etc.*
Sample	*Coffee*	*2 cups*	✓✓	⊙ sm ○ med ○ lg	○ sm ⊙ med ○ lg	Yes (No)	*Running*
6–7 a.m.				○ ○ ○ sm med lg	○ ○ ○ sm med lg	Yes No	
7–8 a.m.				○ ○ ○	○ ○ ○	Yes No	
8–9 a.m.				○ ○ ○	○ ○ ○	Yes No	
9–10 a.m.				○ ○ ○	○ ○ ○	Yes No	
10–11 a.m.				○ ○ ○	○ ○ ○	Yes No	
11–12 noon				○ ○ ○	○ ○ ○	Yes No	
12–1 p.m.				○ ○ ○	○ ○ ○	Yes No	
1–2 p.m.				○ ○ ○	○ ○ ○	Yes No	
2–3 p.m.				○ ○ ○	○ ○ ○	Yes No	
3–4 p.m.				○ ○ ○	○ ○ ○	Yes No	
4–5 p.m				○ ○ ○	○ ○ ○	Yes No	
5–6 p.m.				○ ○ ○	○ ○ ○	Yes No	
6–7 p.m.				○ ○ ○	○ ○ ○	Yes No	

Use this sheet as a master for making copies that you can use as a bladder diary for as many days as you need.

Time	Drinks		Trips to the Bathroom		Accidental Leaks	Did you feel a strong urge to go?	What were you doing at the time?
	What kind?	*How much?*	*How many times?*	*How much urine? (circle one)*	*How much? (circle one)*	*Circle one*	*Sneezing, exercising having sex, lifting, etc.*
Sample	Soda	2 cans	✓✓	⊙ ○ ○ sm med lg	⊙ ○ ○ sm med lg	Yes (No)	**Running**
7–8 p.m.				○ ○ ○	○ ○ ○	Yes No	
8–9 p.m.				○ ○ ○	○ ○ ○	Yes No	
9–10 p.m.				○ ○ ○	○ ○ ○	Yes No	
10–11 p.m.				○ ○ ○	○ ○ ○	Yes No	
11–12 midnight				○ ○ ○	○ ○ ○	Yes No	
12–1 a.m.				○ ○ ○	○ ○ ○	Yes No	
1–2 a.m.				○ ○ ○	○ ○ ○	Yes No	
2–3 a.m.				○ ○ ○	○ ○ ○	Yes No	
3–4 a.m.				○ ○ ○	○ ○ ○	Yes No	
4–5 a.m.				○ ○ ○	○ ○ ○	Yes No	
5–6 a.m.				○ ○ ○	○ ○ ○	Yes No	

I used _____ pads today. I used _____ diapers today (write number).

Questions to ask my health care team: _____

_____

_____

_____

_____

Let's Talk About Bladder Control for Women is a public health awareness campaign conducted by the National Kidney and Urologic Diseases Information Clearinghouse (NKUDIC), an information dissemination service of the National Institute of Diabetes and Digestive and Kidney Diseases (NIDDK), National Institutes of Health.

Kegel Exercise Tips

What are Kegel exercises?

To do Kegel exercises, you just squeeze your pelvic floor muscles. The part of your body including your hip bones is the pelvic area. At the bottom of the pelvis, several layers of muscle stretch between your legs. The muscles attach to the front, back, and sides of the pelvic bone.

Kegel exercises are designed to make your pelvic floor muscles stronger. These are the muscles that hold up your bladder and help keep it from leaking.

Building up your pelvic muscles with Kegel exercises can help with your bladder control.

How do you exercise your pelvic muscles?

Find the right muscles. Try one of the following ways to find the right muscles to squeeze.

1. Imagine that you are trying to stop passing gas. Squeeze the muscles you would use. If you sense a "pulling" feeling, you are squeezing the right muscles for pelvic exercises.

2. Imagine that you are sitting on a marble and want to pick up the marble with your vagina. Imagine "sucking" the marble into your vagina.

3. Lie down and put your finger inside your vagina. Squeeze as if you were trying to stop urine from coming out. If you feel tightness on your finger, you are squeezing the right pelvic muscles.

Let your doctor, nurse, or therapist help you. Many people have trouble finding the right muscles. Your doctor, nurse, or therapist can check to make sure you are doing the exercises correctly. You can also exercise by using special weights or biofeedback. Ask your health care team about these exercise aids.

Don't squeeze other muscles at the same time. Be careful not to tighten your stomach, legs, or other muscles. Squeezing the wrong muscles can put more pressure on your bladder control muscles. Just squeeze the pelvic muscle. Don't hold your breath.

Repeat, but don't overdo it. At first, find a quiet spot to practice— your bathroom or bedroom—so you can concentrate. Lie on the floor. Pull in the pelvic muscles and hold for a count of 3. Then relax for a count of 3. Work up to 10 to 15 repeats each time you exercise. Use the Exercise Log on the other side of this sheet to keep track of your sessions.

Do your pelvic exercises at least three times a day. Every day, use three positions: lying down, sitting, and standing. You can exercise while lying on the floor, sitting at a desk, or standing in the kitchen. Using all three positions makes the muscles strongest.

Be patient. Don't give up. It's just 5 minutes, three times a day. You may not feel your bladder control improve until after 3 to 6 weeks. Still, most women do notice an improvement after a few weeks.

Week: _____

My Pelvic Muscle Exercise Log
Sunday • I exercised my pelvic muscles ____ times. • I spent ____ minutes exercising. • At each exercise session, I squeezed my pelvic muscles ____ times.
Monday • I exercised my pelvic muscles ____ times. • I spent ____ minutes exercising. • At each exercise session, I squeezed my pelvic muscles ____ times.
Tuesday • I exercised my pelvic muscles ____ times. • I spent ____ minutes exercising. • At each exercise session, I squeezed my pelvic muscles ____ times.
Wednesday • I exercised my pelvic muscles ____ times. • I spent ____ minutes exercising. • At each exercise session, I squeezed my pelvic muscles ____ times.
Thursday • I exercised my pelvic muscles ____ times. • I spent ____ minutes exercising. • At each exercise session, I squeezed my pelvic muscles ____ times.
Friday • I exercised my pelvic muscles ____ times. • I spent ____ minutes exercising. • At each exercise session, I squeezed my pelvic muscles ____ times.
Saturday • I exercised my pelvic muscles ____ times. • I spent ____ minutes exercising. • At each exercise session, I squeezed my pelvic muscles ____ times.

Use this sheet as a master for making copies that you can use to record your exercises week after week.

Medicines for Bladder Control

Medicines for bladder control generally work by blocking signals that may cause muscle spasms in the bladder. A group of drugs called antispasmodics are usually the first drugs your doctor will consider for treating bladder control problems. Another group of medicines, called tricyclic antidepressants, may be considered, although these drugs are primarily intended to treat depression. Tricyclic antidepressants can calm nerve signals and decrease spasms in the bladder muscles.

Antispasmodics

Other Names for This Medicine	
Brand Name	**Generic Name**
Detrol	tolterodine
Ditropan	oxybutynin chloride
Enablex	darifenacin
Levsin	hyoscyamine
Sanctura	trospium chloride
VESIcare	solifenacin succinate

Extended-release forms of oxybutynin and tolterodine are now available.

Brand Name	**Generic Name**
Detrol LA	tolterodine extended release
Ditropan XL	oxybutynin extended release

Oxybutynin also comes in a patch that may decrease the side effects (see below).

Brand Name	Generic Name
Oxytrol	oxybutynin patch delivery system

Side effects. Antispasmodics can cause your eyes to become sensitive to light. These medicines also keep you from sweating and can cause dry mouth. If you take any of these medicines, you may need to take a few steps to deal with side effects.

- Wear sunglasses if your eyes become more sensitive to light.
- Take care not to become overheated.
- Chew gum or suck on sugarless hard candy to avoid dry mouth.

Tricyclic Antidepressants

Other Names for This Medicine	
Brand Name	**Generic Name**
Elavil	amitriptyline
Pamelor	nortriptyline
Sinequan	doxepin
Tofranil	imipramine

Side effects. Tricyclic antidepressants can cause your vision to blur when you read, dry mouth, constipation, and light-headedness when you stand after sitting.

Antidiuretic

Other Names for This Medicine	
Brand Name	**Generic Name**
DDAVP	desmopressin
DDAVP Nasal Spray	desmopressin
DDAVP Rhinal Tube	desmopressin
DDVP	desmopressin
Stimate Nasal Spray	desmopressin

Desmopressin is a man-made form of a natural hormone that your body makes. The hormone, called antidiuretic hormone (ADH) or vasopressin, directs the kidneys to make less urine. The urine is therefore more concentrated. Desmopressin is not usually prescribed for adult women with overactive bladder or stress incontinence. It is more often used to treat bedwetting in children. It is also used to treat a condition called diabetes insipidus.

Side effects. Desmopressin rarely causes side effects, but you should call your doctor if you have headaches, stomach cramps, nausea, reddening of the skin, a stuffy or runny nose, or pain in the genital area.

Interstitial Cystitis Medicine

Other Names for This Medicine	
Brand Name	**Generic Name**
Elmiron	pentosan polysulfate sodium

Pentosan is approved to treat the symptoms of bladder pain, urinary frequency, and urinary urgency that characterize interstitial cystitis, also known as painful bladder syndrome. Doctors do not know exactly how it works, but one theory is that it may repair defects that might have developed in the lining of the bladder.

Side effects. Pentosan's side effects are limited primarily to minor gastrointestinal discomfort. A small minority of patients experience some hair loss, but hair grows back when they stop taking the drug. Researchers have found no negative interactions between pentosan and other medications.

Your doctor will order regular blood tests to monitor your liver function while you take pentosan.

Because pentosan has not been tested in pregnant women, the manufacturer recommends that it not be used during pregnancy, except in the most severe cases.

> **All drugs—even those sold over the counter—have potential side effects. Patients should always consult a doctor before using any drug for an extended amount of time.**

www.ingramcontent.com/pod-product-compliance
Lightning Source LLC
Chambersburg PA
CBHW080352290526
45791CB00009BA/2844